Intermittent Fasting for Weight Loss

Complete Guide to Transforming Your Body in 15 Days or Less Guaranteed!

Meal Plan Included

VL DeAlexander

ISBN-13: 978-1-7931-2654-2

CONTENTS

CHAPTER 1

INTRODUCTION

Obesity has become a serious problem all over the world. The World Health Organization has recently announced that since the year 1975, the prevalence of obesity has increased by 300%. Over 650 million people are estimated to be obese throughout the world – and up to 1.9 billion people are also estimated to be overweight.

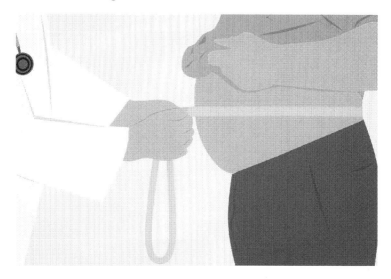

The health risks that obesity carries are serious issues. A number of diseases such as type 2 diabetes, hyperlipidemia, metabolic syndrome, cancer and coronary heart disease, high blood pressure, which can lead to stroke, originate from carrying an excessive amount of body fat. Let's take a look at how obesity has led to some of the diseases mentioned above.

• **Coronary heart disease** - being overweight means that the body mass index (BMI) rises. With obesity, the arteries that supply blood to the heart thicken due to the build-up of a sticky substance called plaque which can hinder blood flow and cause a heart attack.

• **High blood pressure** - the power by which the heart pumps blood through the veins and arteries is known as blood pressure. Obesity causes an increase in this pressure, which leads to many problems in the body over time.

• **Stroke** – obesity, as previously mentioned, causes the formation of plaque. Over time this plaque can cause the formation of blood clots called thrombus. A detached clot causes many serious problems throughout the body: myocardial infarction or heart attack if it lodges in the heart, pulmonary embolism if it travels to the lungs, and stroke if the clot lodges in the brain. Each one is a medical emergency that can be fatal.

• **Abnormal blood fats** – being overweight usually causes an in-crease in bad cholesterol in the body, causing a decrease in good cholesterol. High cholesterol is bad for health and is a risk factor for illness caused by coronary heart disease

Women who are pregnant may also experience problems with their pregnancy due to the complications that obesity causes them to experience.

To address the worldwide prevalence of obesity, a significant number of diets, supplements, and programs have been released. These programs aim to help obese individuals lose the excess weight they have gained, with the hopes of restoring their optimal health. While some of these diets have shown impressive results, even when studied in clinical trials, many do not work, cause people to gain more weight in the long run, and even lead to side-effects.

Intermittent fasting is a type of lifestyle change that many people have adopted recently. Many tend to confuse this "lifestyle option" with a diet – it is not exactly a diet that a person needs to follow, but rather a way of eating – scheduling of food consumption is the most important part of this lifestyle plan.

Here, we will introduce you to intermittent fasting. We'll consider what intermittent fasting really is, the different types of this "dietary" or "life-style" option that is available, how it works, and we will, of course, also consider the benefits and possible drawbacks that everyone should be aware of before setting out to implementing this "eating pattern" into their lives.

CHAPTER 2

UNDERSTANDING INTERMITTENT FASTING

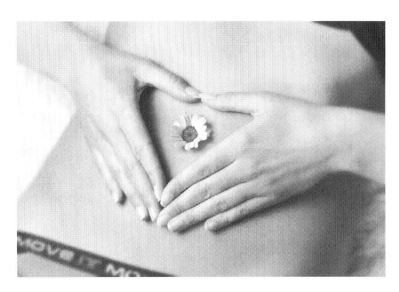

Let us start by taking a look at what intermittent fasting is. The term has become quite popular in recent years, but there is still a lot of confusion in regards to what this term really means and what it involves. Many people think that the term "intermittent fasting" refers to a diet, but this not actually a diet. Instead, it is rather an eating habit that people adopt that gives them guidance on when they should eat – this allows the digestive system to take a break from processing and digesting food continuously.

For many people, this type of dietary habit seems unhealthy. There is a lot of people who are scared of adopting this pattern of eating because they think that they would starve themselves. This, however, is a com-mon myth that has been told about intermittent fasting.

This particular dietary scheduling technique has been used since ancient times. Numerous scientific studies have been conducted to determine how the technique interacts with the human body, and several ad-vantages have already been noted.

An important fact that you should know when it comes to discussing this method of eating is that, since it is not classified as a diet, it will not decide the types of food that you will be eating. It is up to you to decide what you want to eat. A healthy, balanced diet that is filled with foods high in essential nutrients will, of course, result in more benefits as com-pared to stuffing yourself with hamburgers and pizza as soon as the clock strikes five, or whatever time it is your eating cycle starts. When opting for fast foods and other food options that are very high in carbohydrates, weight loss may not be a particular benefit that you experience when following this diet.

Why Do People Use Intermittent Fasting?

There are many different reasons why people use the intermittent fasting technique. These techniques date back to ancient times – they were used historically for a number of different purposes. For example, in older times, when a village would be limited to their food supply, people in the village would often implementing a type of fasting technique to help make the food last longer. Careful planning had to go into such a technique as the villagers had to eat enough food to support their bodily functions, at the right times, while still ensuring the inventory of available food could last until more food would become available.

Certain religions also have certain celebrations and festivals where people fast. Religions that incorporate fasting include Buddhism, Judaism, Islam, Hinduism, Bahai, Jainism, Raelism, and Sikhism. Certain types of Christian religions also use fasting for various purposes. This includes Catholicism, Orthodoxy, Mormonism, and Protestantism. These religions use fasting in different ways, and the technique serves a different purpose in each religion. Some religions also only utilize parts of these fasting techniques and will not completely eliminate all foods from a per-son's diet for a set period of time.

Many people also tend to go on a fast when they feel sick, whether they have contracted the flu or another type of disease. This is because food does not work well with nausea and vomiting, nor with other types of gastrointestinal symptoms.

In modern times, however, more-and-more people are starting to adopt an intermittent fasting lifestyle – often not because they are sick or be-cause of religious requirements, but rather due to the health benefits that have been associated with this scheduled eating habit.

While weight loss is surely the most popular benefit that tends to be the reason why people usually opt for intermittent fasting, it is important to realize that there are more benefits that can be achieved as well. In particular, it has been found that this technique actually changes certain cells in the body. This, in turn, can cause changes in human growth hormone regulation, insulin regulation, and even improve the body's ability to re-pair cells.

Fasting has also been linked to reductions in low-grade chronic inflammation throughout the body, lower levels of oxidative stress in body tis-sues and cells, as well as potential improvements in a person's cardiovascular health. In turn, this combination of powerful benefits may lead to a longer lifespan – while this has not been proven yet, long-term studies are currently being conducted to see whether these benefits can, in fact, prolong a person's life.

The Science Behind Intermittent Fasting

Understanding how exactly intermittent fasting

work is one of the essential elements that need to be covered before you dive into it and start adopting this method of eating in your own life. By learning more about how it works, you can get a better idea of whether or not this might be a good option for you – and if you would be able to benefit from it truly.

This eating habit basically involves cycles of eating and abstaining from food. There are different techniques and methods that have been introduced over the last few years, so not everyone will follow this lifestyle option in the same way as others. Generally, however, all options that are available involved periods of time where food is consumed, and then periods where the person would completely avoid eating any type of food.

When eating normally, with three meals a day and in-between snacks, the body uses energy from the recently consumed meal first, seeking out carbohydrates (CHO) and sugars, which it prefers to burn before anything else. Without intermittent fasting, normal persons (non-diabetics) insulin sensitivity will be at normal levels, and will detect stored glycogen at "full level." With sufficient blood glucose levels, excess energy will be stored as fat. If this happens on a regular basis, the determinants for the difference in body weight will lie in the level of activity and metabolic rate which slows down with age, resulting in weight gain.

When on intermittent fasting, the body behaves differently when food is present (feasting) and during the period of abstinence (fasting), as com-pared to normal eating. The body produces insulin in response to the presence of food, enabling the body to get the most from them, maximizing nutrients for optimum results. Since eating is confined to a desired set window of 4, 6, or 8 hours, the body will not have a ready source of energy during the fasted state and will tend to extract energy from stored fat rather than from glucose traveling in the blood or glycogen stored in the liver or muscles.

Insulin sensitivity is increased after a fast. We can illustrate this insulin sensitivity by analyzing the cascade of events that take place when such a person eats something. As blood glucose rises, it activates a feedback mechanism which signals the pancreas to send insulin to the site where it is needed. An immediate response serves to lower the blood glucose and prevent its accumulation in the blood, or hyperglycemia. Here, insulin responds with a "now you see it, now you don't" type of mechanism: a sharp peak in response to the rising blood glucose, followed by an immediate decline. This is documented by lower readings of 2-hour postprandial blood glucose and insulin measurements.

Diabetics, on the other hand, suffer from insulin resistance, wherein the pancreas secretes only small bursts of insulin in response to glucose, followed by a slowed decline, resulting in higher 2-hour postprandial blood glucose and insulin measurements.

How You Can Use Intermittent Fasting to Lose Weight

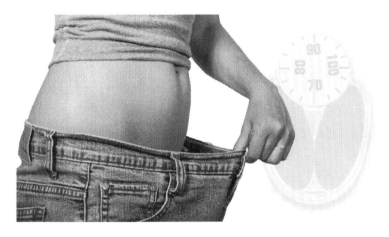

The majority of people who wishes to start implementing intermittent fasting into their lives want to do so due to the weight loss benefits that have been reported. It is well-known by now that this type of eating habit can help a person shed extra weight, primarily through the reduction of calories. Several scientific studies have also been conducted on this topic, and the results have been quite positive thus far. This is why we decided to look at the benefits that intermittent fasting may have for a person who is obese or overweight, and who is currently struggling to lose weight with conventional diets and other types of weight loss programs.

This eating pattern has two particular benefits that should be considered when it comes to losing weight. Firstly, it has been scientifically proven to help shed excess fat. This is a major advantage over traditional diets and dieting supplements – most programs, diets and even the pills that can be taken to initiate weight loss often tend to reduce weight through a reduction in "water weight." Rarely do they truly help a person lose actual fat? With intermittent fasting, however, science has proven that a person burns fat and their body fat percentage becomes reduced when they implement this technique into their lives and strictly stick to the particular routine they have decided on.

The other major benefit in regards to weight loss is that this scheduled eating plan has also been proven to preserve the lean muscle mass in a person's body while they lose weight. This is an important factor that needs to be taken into account. Lean muscle mass is important for several functions of the human body and also helps to make the movement more comfortable.

For example, lean muscle mass has been proven beneficial in the prevention of insulin resistance, as well as diabetes. A loss of lean muscle mass has also been associated with a higher incidence of illness. Cancer patients, for example, who loses muscle mass while undergoing treatment are less likely to survive and more likely to experience a recurrence of the disease should they survive, as compared to those who maintain healthier levels of muscle mass.

Furthermore, research has also been proven that lean muscle mass helps to maintain stronger bones. When bones are kept in a healthy and strong state, then a person is less likely to experience problems such as fragile bones and problems maintaining their balance. The person will also be less likely to suffer an injury during physical activity. The risk of osteoarthritis and similar diseases are also lower among individuals with stronger bones and better levels of lean muscle mass.

Several suggestions have been made regarding the way that intermittent fasting would help a person lose excess fat, while also preserving their existing muscle mass. The effect that these scheduled eating habits have on the body's metabolism is thought to play a significant role here. For example, one review paper explains that the gut flora, often also called the microbiome, is affected by intermittent fasting. This, in turn, can help to improve metabolism and make the digestive system more efficient.

Another study explains that, even though it is widely recognized this that habit of eating based on specific cycles are beneficial for obese individuals, little data is available on how exactly this works on a biological or physiological level. The study found that fat reduction is possible primarily due to adipose thermogenesis that occurs due to the energy or caloric restriction imposes upon a person's body with this type of approach to eating.

Other Possible Benefits of Intermittent Fasting

Besides weight loss, intermittent fasting carries with it many other health benefits, some of which are:

The practice of intermittent fasting is for every individual who is interested in the accrual of health benefits into his life. It is not designed merely for the obese or the out-of-shape clientele. Maintaining optimal health is both a privilege and responsibility of every human being created by God.

Intermittent fasting breeds longevity. Scientific studies have re-ported that this eating pattern results in positive outcomes in favor of improving quality of life. So it is not just staying alive per se, but being able to live and appreciate life fully. Imagine our body as a machine that undergoes wear and tears with the stress of eating, digestion, calorie utilization, delivery to the tissues and elimination of wastes. Intermittent fasting would cut that wear and tear right in the middle, because eating is confined within a personally chosen window, and the body is given a respite from the digestive processes during the fasting period.

Knowing that the human body is never idle, even during rest, and that there is always something going on inside, pathways are activated, signaling the body to quickly grab the opportunity to regenerate, repair and rejuvenate muscles, organs, and tissues, thereby delaying the aging process.

Intermittent fasting has the long-term effect of normalizing insulin sensitivity. This is beneficial because insulin resistance plays a crucial role in the etiology of chronic diseases such as Diabetes Mellitus Type 2, Heart Disease and certain types of cancer.

Intermittent fasting curbs hunger by regulating the level of ghrelin, which is known as the "hunger hormone."

Intermittent fasting activates the Growth Hormone, which plays a pivotal role in overall health and muscle growing fitness.

Intermittent fasting reduces inflammatory conditions and promotes cellular resistance to free radical damage through the process of natural detoxification.

Intermittent fasting normalizes blood pressure and blood lipids.

Intermittent fasting simplifies the daily routine. Mothers no longer have to rush through the morning to prepare breakfast for the family, prepare and hustle the kids off to school, rush to the office if she is a working mom, and the list goes on. This is an interesting benefit that is attributed to intermittent fasting. We only have to plan for 1-2 meals a day depending on your chosen window, ideally composed of 30-35% high-quality chewable protein in the form of meat, 30-35% fat from non-animal sources, and 35-40% complex carbohydrates.

Intermittent fasting lowers the risk of cancer. The development of cancer on a cellular level is encouraged by the quality of food consumed, especially those high in sugars, saturated fat, seasonings, coloring, and preservatives, to name a few. Because intermittent fasting would require a dramatic change not only in the frequency of meals but also in the nutrient content, the body would be less subjected to assault from the toxins from highly processed food and empty calories. With restricted calories, our body has much more time to burn the food and optimize the use of nutrients, using up fat stores which are known to fuel breast and other reproductive organ cancers. Also, high fiber content would serve to mobilize and excrete any present undesirables out of the body. Another important caveat is, that cancer cells feed on sugars, while high fructose, an ingredient which is present in various forms, whether overt or covert, causes cancer cell division.

Intermittent fasting delays the aging process, especially if combined with some form of exercise. Stress resistance is enhanced, reducing oxidative damage up to the cellular level, acting as a deterrent to aging. Increased resistance against free radicals also discourages the development of inflammatory diseases and some forms of cancer. Also, studies have shown that fasting before chemotherapy increases the success rate of the treatment, as evidenced by the destruction of neuroblastoma cells.

Intermittent fasting makes weight loss and muscle building attainable. A majority of people who want to lose weight cannot stick to a diet. Fad diets turn into the latest craze but evaporate into thin air eventually. What's more, long-term use of any of these fad diets can result in serious deficits which yield detrimental effects to one's health. Some diets can result in water retention which can congest the heart; others result in water loss which can lead to dehydration, affecting the balance of sodium and potassium in the body; still, others which advocate an all-protein diet with no carbs can have dire consequences. Weight loss does occur, but has a pendulum or yo-yo effect on the health, the weight loss during the course of the diet is quickly gained back when the regimen is no longer in force. All this creates stress on the heart and organs, not to mention pressure on the part of the dieter to lose weight.

Another problem that many people face has to do with food restrictions. Without fail, these restrictions will become even more appealing and is often a cause for violations. For this reason, intermittent fasting presents a better option as a weight loss program. Some people maintain the notion that the hunger we feel is just a state of mind, and we need to communicate that idea to our bodies. Reality tells us that THIS IS DEFI-NITELY NOT SO! How would you console your hungry tummy, with all its musical growls that feeling hungry is just a state of mind? I cannot imagine how to tell a growling tummy to shut up!

Many people find the idea of fasting for twelve to 24 hours difficult since it involves behavior modification of deeply ingrained eating habits. At the start, there will surely be a transition period from "all the time eating" to "scheduled eating." The idea is to work it up gradually, from your normal eating pattern to an 8 to 10-hour window, then reduce it to 6 to 8 hours and even less if desired. Choose first whether you are going to skip breakfast or dinner and work around it accordingly. Know that it is okay to drink water, green or black tea or black coffee during your fasting period, but don't overdo it. There is no limit to the amount of pure water you can drink; and in fact, out of habit we typically reach for food or a snack when our bodies are actually crying for water instead.

Although difficulties will be encountered, it is the positive results that will be inspiring. Intermittent fasting is not just about overcoming the idea of hunger to be able to go without food for some time. It is more of establishing a new pattern of eating which can yield the desired benefits of weight loss and muscle shaping.

You will be surprised to discover that that **intermittent fasting can provide better mental clarity and concentration.** This is a great benefit of implementing the intermittent fasting pattern of eating be-cause it is important to have days filled with energy and mental clarity. This increases productivity and the creative output and puts you in an excellent mood for the day.

There are also many other benefits of intermittent fasting which involve the sympathetic and parasympathetic nervous system, but none of these benefits will be felt if you are only practicing fasting while sleeping. For best results a person with a highly active lifestyle should implement intermittent fasting for 16 hours; 24-hour fasts are recommended for those with a lower level of activity. This is what the "experts" say, but you don't have to make a drastic move just to find out that it doesn't work for you. I suggest that you make whatever transition slowly according to your own pace, but whatever you do, keep going.

Common Myths and Issues with Intermittent Fasting

Knowing human nature, we have to deal with our fears squarely, especially when it comes to lifestyle changes that veer away from the norms of family and society. Like most, we have been programmed to believe certain ideas to be true, because we have heard it being mouthed by people we respect. Some examples of these are:

Alcohol will fatten you up, so you may not take alcoholic drinks while fasting or on a diet. The truth is that the body has a hard time breaking down ethanol, let alone converting it to fat.

Short-term fasting decreases metabolic rate. Scientific studies show the exact opposite.

Breakfast is the most important meal of the day. The Kellogg Company has bombarded us with advertisements to this effect, so many of us believe that it's "breakfast first thing in the morning." We have heard the same statement from our grandparents and parents, and we could not leave for school without breakfast.

Cooked meals can be replaced by shakes, meal replacement powers, and protein bars. This is the answer to today's busy lifestyle, the coping mechanism of this get-up-and-go generation, but we know better. The oldies know that there is no substitute for sitting down to a nice warm meal.

But many have come to believe it because of

Repetition. We hear it being said over and over,

and since many believe it, then it must be true.

Advertisements. We are constantly bombarded by TV commercials, print, and even pop-ups on our computer.

Knowledge deficit on the part of the general public. We need to educate ourselves, especially on things concerning our health.

There are eight notions (there could be more) which in one way or another may affect public acceptance of the intermittent fasting eating pattern, and these are

NOTION 1: **Fasting or dieting will ruin your metabolism and make you fat and hungry.**

ANSWER: There is a slight increase in metabolic rate in direct proportion to the number of calories consumed.

NOTION 2: **Eat smaller meals more often for hunger control**

ANSWER: It is not so much the frequency of the meal which will control hunger. If the meal is made up of carbohydrates and simple sugars, the body will burn these quickly and be hungry again in a short time. Moreover, if the body expects to be fed every few hours, there would be no motivation to seek other fuels to burn; add to that little or no activity, and the excess calories are stored as fat. Three high-protein balanced meals control appetite better than six high-protein meals. Aside from the change in composition, it would be wise to cut down on caloric density and increasing volume by replacing with cruciferous vegetables and complex carbohydrates.

NOTION 3: **Eat small meals regularly to keep blood sugar under control and provide an alert mind and energetic body.**

ANSWER: Blood sugar follows the meal pattern you are accustomed to. In normal individuals, blood sugar is naturally stable. In those with insulin resistance, stability is subject to the usual diet, food intake, hormone-regulated patterns, and hereditary factors.

There is no need to eat regularly to control blood sugar levels since blood sugar is able to maintain itself and adjusts to your chosen eating pattern,

NOTION 4: **Fasting switches the body gears into "starvation mode."**

ANSWER: After a meal, the body's metabolic rate increases and remains so until 60 hours after. There is no decrease in metabolic rate that occurs until after 60 hours of fasting. Therefore, to say that the body switches to "starvation mode" as a result of fasting is not true.

NOTION 5: **Consume proteins every 2-3 hours to maintain a steady supply of amino acids.**

ANSWER: This eating pattern would put the body under great stress. It takes more than 5 hours for the body to digest a standard meal, and amino acids are still being released into the blood and absorbed by muscles until much later. It all depends on the meal composition, such as a type of protein, carbohydrates, fiber and what was ingested during prior meals. These are the factors that determine how long amino acids will be made available to the tissues after meals. So after 5 hours, you are still "anabolic," essentially meaning that the energy from your food is still accessible for tissue growth and maintenance.

NOTION 6: **Fasting causes muscle loss.**

ANSWER: Just by changing meal frequency, the effect of regular fasting on muscle contour showed the fat loss and increased muscle gain even without changing calorie intake or weight training. The issue of catabolism does not become a problem with short-term controlled fasting. The body would not enter into a catabolic state, a condition that is mainly caused by excessive training in conjunction with inadequate protein nutrition unless there is impaired protein absorption coupled with long fasting periods daily. And this happens gradually when amino acids are not available from food, and stored liver glycogen is depleted.

NOTION 7: **Skipping breakfast is bad and will make you fat.**

ANSWER: Breakfast skippers are seen as those who engage in crash diets, have higher weight and BMI. After a fasting period through sleep, insulin sensitivity is highest in the morning, increased after glycogen depletion, and breakfast eater's exhibit better controls over their dietary habits. This is what made people think that breakfast is healthy and improves insulin sensitivity. Recent studies show otherwise.

NOTION 8: **Fasting increases cortisol.**

ANSWER: Cortisol increases in response to a stressor, to help the body's stress coping mechanism.

This is related to the breakfast issue, in that breakfast eaters suffer post-breakfast hunger which is triggered by an in-crease in cortisol levels following an all-night fast; and misinterpreting these body signals triggers and all-day eating pattern. This increased cortisol level has benefits, which is why it was suggested to exercise early in the morning on an empty stomach because one can maintain an adequate rate of exertion for a long time without suffering pain, hunger, and fatigue. Cortisol increases wakefulness, alertness and memory recall. So used in conjunction with fasting, it has good effects. Bad effects will hap-pen if the exposure to a stressor is prolonged.

When we are accustomed to eating many times per day, the feeling of hunger in our body will normally cause panic, and we start looking for food. But, what happens if we don't get to consume that food? Absolutely nothing. Our health won't be threatened by missing a few meals.

There is a difference between psychological and physical hunger. When we feel hungry, the psychological hunger is present. We just think that we are hungry, but our body has enough fuel to function well. At this time, our body is burning the fat deposits, and we are slimming down. Some-times, eating is done out of habit and is a result of our thoughts. When we see a food commercial, we are psychologically stimulated to feel hunger, even if we have eaten an hour barely before.

By using intermittent fasting, we are putting our bodies and minds into a self-imposed rest period for a determined period of time. For some people, this period is simply the sleeping time. Interesting, right? If the last consumed meal is at eight pm, and the next time we eat is at eight am, there are twelve hours during which our body is fasting. Other people are deciding for some different type of fasting. For example, one meal is in the afternoon, and the next meal is consumed the next afternoon at the same time. You are probably wondering how this can be healthy and help you gain muscle. Well, it actually is. There have been many studies and experiments conducted on this subject that prove this is the healthiest way to lose surplus weight. The data collected by all of the research shows that with proper usage of intermittent fasting, people could extend the length of their life, regulate their blood pressure, regulate weight and easily gain lean muscle with exercise.

Simply put, intermittent fasting is not a magical formula which guarantees immediate results. It takes discipline and a conscious decision to follow through. But if you are new to intermittent fasting, take heart. If you decide that breakfast is the meal to skip, but on one of those days you feel like you need a break, go ahead and do it. Make your experience with intermittent fasting fun and exciting.

CHAPTER 3

TYPES OF INTERMITTENT FASTING

Several different methods can be tailored to individual needs and preferences. There are many familiar methods, but five of them are the most commonly used. It is not important which one is the most used or most desired by others, and it is important to find the method that works best for you and makes your life easier, which in turn make it easier to stick to this practice. Below is a brief overview of each of the five most commonly chosen methods for starting intermittent fasting.

The Daily Method, Also Known as Leangains

Initially introduced by Martin Berkhan, the Leangains method is a practice where fasting is performed for a 14 to 16 hour period and then allows a six to eight-hour window for eating. While the fasting period is on, you are not allowed to consume any calories. Of course, black coffee and sugar-free gum can be consumed, but it is better to stick to only pure water. For most people, this method is the best one because it allows them to enter into the routine easily and to see results faster. The period chosen for fasting can be during the night so that during some period of the day meals are allowed so that hunger won't discourage you so easily.

As mentioned before, fasting as a method can help to burn fat, but also to gain muscle instead of losing. To get the most from this method and get those sexy muscles, the kind of food you eat during the allowed feeding period is very important. It is well known that muscles are made in the kitchen, so let's see what is better to eat and when it is best to eat it. When working out, our body needs carbs to have the strength to with-stand the effort that exercising takes. The intake of protein should be on a high level, mostly every day depending on the gender, age, and fitness activity, in opposition to fats, which are allowed a higher intake only on the days when you are not exercising.

Martin Berkhan provides a few guidelines for those who are trying to gain muscle while practicing this method. According to him, on workout days there should be three meals eaten. If the first meal is close enough to the workout, it should include some carbs. The meal after the workout should be the largest meal eaten during the whole day, and you can include some dessert such as ice cream or maybe a piece of cheesecake. When you have a rest day, the calories consumed should be less than calories consumed on the workout day. On a rest day, the first meal should be your largest meal and should include a higher level of protein. There are also many other things to share, but these are the basics that will help you to get those lean muscles.

The Warrior Method

Introduced by Ori Hofmekler, the warrior diet is a fasting method that people who can follow the rules will be happy to put into practice. This diet works with twenty hours of fasting followed by one big meal. Eating a big meal is probably the key to this method. While the fasting period is on, you are able to have some fruit or vegetables, in low amounts of course. The permitted food intake is not at all a coincidence in this meth-od. Fresh food will increase the work of the nervous system by stimulating adrenaline that will contribute to fat burning. An interesting fact about this method is that the intake of food into the body only takes place during the nighttime hours, which subdues the nervous system and al-lows the spending of calories and improves the digestive process.

Another interesting thing is that this period provides relaxation and growth of muscles in the body. But, this can be misunderstood by some-one. Using this method, you should not expect to gain muscle as with the other methods, mainly because of the fact that food is limited to one meal during the night.

Of course, many people may find this way of losing weight pretty hard. Taking the main meal at night can be a serious problem for some people. Starvation throughout the day can also be a serious obstacle to overcome while practicing this method. But if someone has decided to practice it, they will endure throughout all of this.

Alternately Eating: Eat Stop Eat

Started by Brad Pilon, this method of fasting helps many people to lose weight and to boost their body. The concept behind this method is based on the following: you can eat everything you want during the week, except for one or two days when you shouldn't eat anything for 24 hours. As long as this period of fasting lasts, you can consume water, as well as some calorie-free drinks. The reason why some people find this method the perfect one for them is that they don't need to stay away from the things they want to eat; by fasting one or two days per week, they are lowering their calorie intake for the whole week, so they will manage to lose weight.

Even this method can be difficult for some people, but as its creator says, it is very efficient. It is a method that is flexible, and you can obtain the benefits of it as fast as you want. If you are not ready to put yourself in a fasting mode for whole 24 hours, you can start with as much time as you can manage to begin with and gradually increase the hours until you reach 24 hours. As with the first method, it is recommended to do some type of training, such as resistance training, so your body can burn fat and discover those lean, formed muscles much more quickly.

Fat Loss Forever Method

The fat loss forever method is an intermittent fasting method in cheating is allowed. This may be a great thing for people who like to lose weight but cannot stick to some strict diet or the hours of fasting that the other methods require. This method is actually a hybrid method created by Dan Go and John Romaniello, eliminating all the weaknesses that can be faced when practicing other methods. This program is often practiced for twelve weeks, in which one day per week you are allowed to cheat, and right after this day comes the 36 hours of fasting. This last number will scare most of us, right? The creators of this method suggest performing the fasting on the busiest days of the week, so we won't have a lot of time to think of food.

In addition to this method, there is a training program that can aid in gaining muscle and losing even more weight. Many people may find this method difficult, especially those who are not accustomed to fasting. The cheat days could be threatening to some in the sense that during these days they could consume much more food than they normally would. But everything is in the self-control, isn't it?

Alternate Day Fasting

Alternate day fasting, also known as the Up Day, Down Day Diet, was created by James Johnson and is based on a simple philosophy. You should eat less for one day, and the next day you should eat as you normally do. This "less" means that during the fasting day, the calorie intake should be about 400 to 500 calories less than the days when you eat normally. For gaining muscle, exercising is recommended during the normal calorie days, since on low-calorie days you may find exercising difficult which could lead to discouragement.

This method is probably the easiest method to follow. But, what could happen with the usage of this method is that people may transform their normal calorie day into a lower calorie day, not noticing that it can cause them to challenge the results obtained with this way of fasting. Precisely for this reason, if this method is chosen, it is a good idea to plan in advance the meals for the next day in order to keep the level of calories within the desired frame.

Practicing intermittent fasting is a great way to learn how to control hunger and get in shape easy and fast. Using some of the methods mentioned above, you can easily stick to the fasting and maintain the fast for the de-sired length of time. The best thing that people can learn by practicing fasting is to control the hunger and recognize it for what it is. There are many examples that prove that this practice can lead to weight loss and building muscle.

CHAPTER 4

LOSING WEIGHT WITH INTERMITTENT FASTING

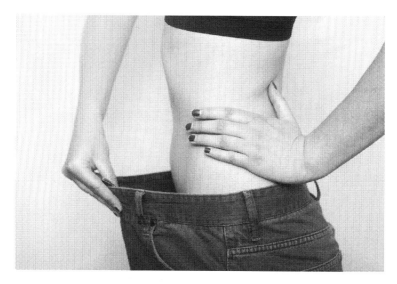

Weight loss is one of the most important reasons why people implement an intermittent fasting program in their lives. The weight loss benefits of this eating plan have been proven – in addition to assisting with metabolism, the diet also helps to curb your appetite, which means you will eat less.

With intermittent fasting, it is essential that you understand it is possible to gain weight instead of to lose weight if your diet is not appropriate. You will need to implement an appropriate diet in order to ensure that you achieve a caloric deficit, while still providing your body with the essential nutrients it relies on daily to perform all of the functions that are crucial to your own survival.

Different types of meal plans have been suggested for those people who are looking to lose weight through intermittent fasting. In the end, it is up to you to choose a meal plan that is appropriate for you. You will have to take yourself into account – consider how much weight you have to lose, and take into account any particular health conditions that you may be suffering from. These will all help you determine how many calories you should consume on a daily basis, how active you will need to be, and what types of food you will be able to include in your intermittent fasting diet plan.

The first step to losing weight with this type of eating habit would be to select an appropriate type of intermittent fasting program. We have al-ready discussed the various options out there that you can select from. Most people find that the standard 16/8 intermittent fasting program is ideal for them if they are only getting started. You can vary the number of days during the week that you will be following this program – some are also able to follow through with the 16/8 program for the entire week. You'll essentially have to listen to your own body – when you feel that you are starving yourself too much, adjust your plan in order to make up for the excessive reduction in your daily caloric consumption. On the other hand, if you find that you are not losing weight, it might be a good idea to take a look at your calorie balance – how much calories are you consuming and how much are you burning through physical activity?

Example Meal Plan for Weight Loss with Intermittent Fasting

If you do a quick search on Google for a weight loss plan that you can use with intermittent fasting, you will be surprised at just how many variations there are that you can choose from. This can really make the entire process challenging, instead of a fun and exciting journey that you are taking on in order to help you achieve a body that you will feel more confident about.

Many of the weight loss plans available can be effective if you stick to the plan and you ensure your body is provided with an adequate amount of exercise on a daily basis. Unfortunately, this does not make it easier to choose one that is ideal for yourself.

Below, we will take a look at an example of a really good intermittent fasting diet plan that you can follow and adjust according to your own preferences and requirements if you are finding it hard to choose an appropriate option for yourself. This is a very basic "framework" that you can work from.

Before we look at the example weight loss intermittent fasting meal plan – there is one thing that you should note. DO not expect everything to go smoothly the first time around. On your first few days, know that things can be rather difficult. This is especially true if you are used to eating continuously during the day – which is a very common problem among people who have a more significant amount of weight to lose.

Be patient in the beginning – with yourself and with the results you achieve through your diet plan. After a week or two, if you do not see the results that you expect, then aim to make a few adjustments in order to customize your diet plan and your intermittent fasting program to be more appropriate to your goals.

With the diet plan example that I am about to share with you – I want you to get into a habit of skipping breakfast. With the 16/8 program, you will only have a window between six to eight hours where you will consume food every day. Since you are aiming to lose weight, skipping out on breakfast means your body will start to utilize its own fat reserves in or-der to generate energy. This is ideal for someone who needs to lose weight.

You will have your first meal at 3 pm in the afternoon. Have your second meal at around 6 pm and then finish off the day with a final meal at around 10 pm.

Your first two meals of the day should be kept

light. This way, you won't turn off your body's automatic fat burning mechanisms. By the end of the day, you'll consume a meal that is heavier on the calorie side. Even though you are free to experiment with the number of calories you consume during each meal, be wary of what food you decide to consume – you are trying to lose weight and become a healthier person. For this rea-son, always ensure that you eat healthily as well.

I personally recommend that the first two meals of your day should be a maximum of 400 calories each. Be sure that there is an adequate supply of protein in these meals. Don't skim on vegetables and fruits – enjoy them as they are good for you.

Here are some examples of small and light meals that you may wish to experiment with for your first two meals (at 3 pm and at 6 pm):

• Add some almonds and a couple of berries into a cup of Greek yogurt.
• Have some cottage cheese with a couple of almonds.
• Add one tablespoon of olive oil to a can of tuna, and enjoy your meal with an apple.
• Use two whole eggs to make yourself an omelet. Have this meal with some delicious berries.

If you are in the mood for a meatier meal, then cook up a chicken breast and enjoy it with a green salad. You can add half of an Avocado to the meal, as well as an apple.

For those who are in a hurry and would like to drink something instead, mixing a cup of unsweetened almond milk with about 40 grams of whey protein powder is a really good option. You can have some fruit with this, as well as about 20 grams of almonds.

When it comes to the third meal of the day – this is when you should enter the kitchen and prepare something healthy and delicious-tasting for yourself. There are a lot of different healthy meals that you can choose to fill the gap at 10 pm. It is a good idea to limit the last meal of the day to around 800 calories, but you can push it up to around 1000 calories if you wish.

When it comes to your last meal, it is important to balance fats and protein perfectly to avoid weight gain or other potential side-effects from your diet plan. If you are opting for a leaned piece of meat (to supply your body with quality protein), then you can have more healthy types of fats in your meal. If, on the other hand, you decide to opt for a fattier type of meal, let's say a piece of beef steak that is a fatty cut, then you should limit how much-added fats you put into your meal.

To help you prepare your third and final meal of the day, here are three examples of meals that are nutritious and will give you that final amount of calories that you need during your eating window:

• Cook up a chicken breast and serve it with some potato wedges and a variety of vegetables.

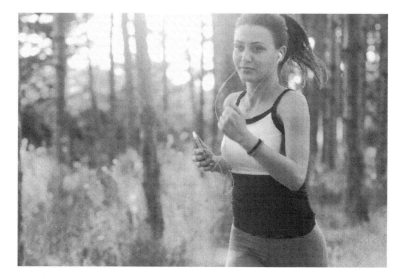

• Serve some brown rice with vegetables and a chicken breast. Try to use a small amount of coconut oil to cook both the rice and the chicken.

• If you are rather in the mood for some beef, then have a steak with some vegetables. You can also serve this up with a sweet potato – add a little bit of cinnamon to the sweet potato for additional flavor.

Exercising with Intermittent Fasting

Ask anyone who had successful results with any type of dieting program in the past – and they would tell you that exercise was a crucial part of their weight loss program. The primary idea behind any type of diet that aims to help you reduce your body weight is to create a caloric deficit. A caloric deficit simply means the number of calories you burn each day through your exercise protocols are higher than the number of calories you consume, as we have already discussed.

Thus, when you are implementing a diet plan along with intermittent fasting to help you lose weight, then you should ensure that you also implement an appropriate exercise program.

Some people are concerned about exercising while following a program that utilizes intermittent fasting strategies. However, once your body is used to this new eating style, you'll notice that it becomes easier and easier. There are also a variety of supplements that you can take to boost your endurance and stamina and to give you that extra energy that you will need to ensure you can get past a training session, even while you are fasting.

Here's a little-known secret that many people do not realize in terms of exercising while you are on an intermittent fasting program: the fat burning mechanisms of the human body is regulated by what is known as the sympathetic nervous system. This system is also called the SNS for short. When the system activates, it means your body starts to burn fat. There are two essential elements that cause the SNS system to activate – this includes a lack of food in your body, as well as exercise. When you decide to give your body a dose of both, then activation is more thorough, and your SNS will lead to a much more significant level of fat burning and weight loss.

There are many other benefits that should be taken into account in terms of exercising while you are fasting. One particular benefit that becomes especially useful for those people who are trying to bulk up with muscle mass while they are following a plan that uses intermittent fasting is the fact that exercising during your fast window will cause oxidative stress. While oxidative stress is often considered a bad thing for the body, during exercise, it can actually be good for improving your muscle strength and mass.

Take this into account as well – if you eat before you participate in an exercise program, then there is a chance that the food you consumed may lead to issues with your general performance during your routine. It has been found that the consumption of food in any form – be it a shake, an energy bar, or an actual meal – causes your blood glucose levels to experience a spike while you are exercising. Sure, this will give you some energy to kickstart that tough routine that you are about to start – but, once this spike is over, your blood glucose levels will quickly decline, and you will basically experience a "crash." What this means is you will feel the fatigue coming on quickly, leading to poor muscle performance and a body that is quickly running out of energy.

There are, however, some publications that say this is a myth – but this is still something that you should consider when it comes to intermittent fasting!

All-in-all, there is a specific number of benefits that you may expect from a good workout program integrated into your intermittent fasting plan. You will be able to experience the following potential benefits with this particular combination:

• You can turn back what is known as the

"biological clock" on your brain, as well as your muscles, due to the effects of exercise on your body while in a fasting state.

• The concentration of growth hormone produced by your body will be increased.

• Your body composition will be greatly improved, as you will experience a reduction in body fat percentage, along with an increase in lean muscle mass.

• Cognitive function will also benefit, and you'll find that problems like brain fog start to disappear.

• Your testosterone levels are likely to rise as well, which can be especially beneficial for older men who are experiencing a natural de-cline in the level of circulating testosterone within their bodies.

While exercising while fasting is definitely beneficial for you and your weight, there is one particular factor that I have to mention here. On days when you are going to do some heavy lifting as part of your exercise routine, it is crucial that you get your timing right. When you decide to participate in some heavy lifting exercises, then you will need to ensure you eat something within the first 30 minutes after you have completed the heavy lifting workout.

CHAPTER 5

CAN YOU BUILD LEAN MUSCLE WITH INTERMITTENT FASTING?

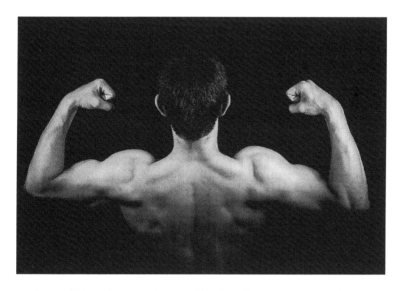

Practicing intermittent fasting has a proven impact on reducing body weight. Of course, the practice of exercising is an additional way to re-duce weight and is important not only when fasting, but always because it helps us to protect and maintain our general health. When following a fasting method, it is better to stick to some type of plan which can pro-vide even better results. Many are reluctant to accept this way of eating, when their main purpose is to create muscle, knowing that in the world of fitness getting a muscular body requires a very different diet. Fasting might seem daunting to many knowing that you should not eat for a period of approximately 16 hours of daylight, depending on the method chosen to be practiced. But when you consider that we spend eight hours in bed, and you go by the rule of no eating at least two hours before going to bed, you can easily endure an additional five to eight hours of fasting.

Below are some guidelines that can help you get the best results from intermittent fasting.

When fasting, try low-intensity cardio. When fasting, our body receives fewer calories during that meal than what is allowed. With fewer received calories, high-intensity cardio exercises can cause the opposite effect. Our body will show us what intensity is sufficient, beginning to experience shortness of breath is a sign that we need to stick to that intensity.

Try to exercise a few hours after you've eaten. After you consume a meal, the body begins to break down fats, sugars, carbohydrates, etc. In return, the body releases glycogen which acts as fuel for the body during exercise. At the same time, this way removes the risk of lowering blood sugar which will make us feel weak and exhausted if its levels become too low.

The entry of large amounts of protein will put you closer to your goal. To be able to put into practice the intermittent fasting and also build a strong and well-muscled body during the time in which eating is allowed, you need to consume greater amounts of protein. The exact timing of the intake of proteins which, along with carbohydrates, should be a few hours before exercise as well as after the completion of the exercise, will help make it easier to complete the training and build the de-sired muscle.

It is good to include snacks throughout the day. If the method you selected for fasting time allows, the intake of snacks during certain time periods will help blood sugar levels to remain normal. By maintaining normal blood sugar levels, we can have the energy to be able to practice the exercises properly and do more repetitions which will contribute to the combustion of a large quantity of fat.

Although perhaps this practice will run into some of the mistrust, if the food is consumed properly, the muscles can be easily built. The first thing that should be done for successful implementation of occasional fasting in the process of building muscle is to determine the level of required calories for your body. This course is individual and different for every person. After you determine the required amount of calories, you need to decide on a pre-workout to take around twenty percent of total daily calories. This dish should be eaten just before the workout and need to contain sufficient carbs which will certainly give energy and proteins which are essential for muscle growth. The rest of the required daily calories should be distributed through the rest of the time after a workout while fasting has not started. This may involve a lot of food for many, especially if training is late in the afternoon, but with the right choice of food, calories will certainly help. The way the occasional fasting helps in terms of building muscle is that after the training the body needs carbo-hydrates to help regain strength; the intake of large amounts of fat can be harmful in these moments. Precisely for this reason, you can choose a larger meal containing carbs and protein, which allows the combination of fat and protein to remain for several hours after training, in order to reduce the need for carbohydrates in large quantities.

Stay hydrated

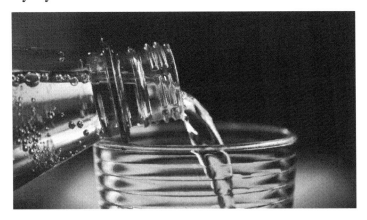

We all are aware that 95% of our body is made up of water. The introduction of a certain amount of water, from 1.5L to 3L depending on the individual, is important not only for the occasional practice of fasting but al-so for maintaining health in everyday life. But the reason I mention this is not just that. It is because with the consumption of water, we suppress hunger and it is easier to deal with methods that are designed for fasting.

Water is important for balancing the body's different systems such as the heart, brain, kidneys, lungs and of course, the biggest one, muscles. On the other hand, the intake of the required amount of water is important because the muscles need water for moisture and growth. Water is also important because we flex and move our muscles. If we do not drink enough water during the day, our body will become dehydrated, and muscle control and strength will be impaired. With the proper amount of water, we can easily build strong muscles and get the best results from the training. Dehydration will also lead to unhealthy, sagging skin and slower muscle response.

Measure the results and stay motivated

Seeing results always give the greatest motivation. In terms of weight loss, it can often be disappointing if we do not begin to see the results of our efforts quickly. That is the reason why many people try to reduce excess weight before starting. The practice of occasional fasting gives visible results in a short period of time if properly practiced.

The results that occasionally gives can be quite impressive. With proper usage of certain exercises, (depending on the purpose of the current training, or whether our goal is to create a lithe body with lean muscles or a body with large, defined muscles) muscles will gradually increase, pushing out the fat, until they become visible. What must be noted is that you should not rely on scales, for the simple reason that weight is increased due to the building of muscle, which weighs more than fat. The best way to monitor results is with images. Before the occasional fasting combined with the training that you alone will determine, take a picture of yourself and remember the date. Each subsequent week or month, take a new photograph, and you will be amazed when you see how your body is changing. Each week your muscle will be hidden by less fat deposits.

CHAPTER 6

DEVELOPING AN INTERMITTENT FASTING MEAL PLAN

Once you have decided to start with an intermittent fasting program – whether it is to help you lose weight and get healthier or to take ad-vantage of other health benefits that have been associated with this eating style – you will need to go through a phase where you will plan for the big change that is coming up. You'll have to choose the type of intermit-tent fasting plan you would like to follow, and you need to decide how you will be implementing this type of eating plan into your own life.

It is important to not just jump into intermittent fasting without planning out how you will go about your new diet plan first. Without a solid plan, you might end up cheating, eating the wrong foods, or doing things in such a wrong way that you may experience serious side effects from your new diet.

One of the most important things that you need to target when you are planning out your intermittent fasting program would be the meal plan. Most people find that it is much easier to continue following an intermit-tent fasting program if they know what they will have for dinner or what snacks they should pack for when that time comes when they can start catching up on the time they spent committed to fasting.

For some people, it can be difficult to set up a meal plan that will be effective. It is essential, as described already, to ensure a meal plan fits in with the specific goals that you might be striving for with intermittent fasting.

Before you can start to plan out your meals while you are going to be following an intermittent fasting program, make sure that you know exactly what your goals are and why are you planning to implement this pro-gram. Do you want to lose weight? Would you like to build muscle at the same time? Are you simply looking to try out intermittent fasting for other types of benefits? Your goals will ultimately help you set up a meal plan that will allow you to reach them and to take advantage of what intermittent fasting is able to offer you.

In addition to considering the goals that you are striving toward with intermittent fasting, you will also need to take into account the type of intermittent fasting program that you will be following. Some allow you to eat for specified times during the day, and others require fasting for the major part of the day. There are different options available – and we have already looked at the options that you can choose from.

Since there are so many varieties of intermittent fasting to choose from, we would really need a completely separate book to look at every type of meal plan that you could develop in order to set up an appropriate plan for your journey. To make things simpler, we will take a look at one or two examples of meal plans that you could follow. This will give you an idea of what to expect, what type of foods to include, and more.

Examples of Meal Plans for 16/8 Intermittent Fasting Option

Example #1

Let's start by taking a look at a meal plan for the 16/8 intermittent fasting model. With this particular option, you would fast for 16 hours of the day and then enjoy eight hours where you are allowed to eat. The following is just a simple example of a meal plan – you can take from it and make appropriate modifications in order to include the foods that you require to achieve your goal.

You would start the day with a fresh cup of black coffee – no milk or creamer, and absolutely no sugar. This will help to give your digestive system and metabolism a good kickstart for the day, without adding calories to your day.

Coffee has a host of benefits for your body, which

is why it is a great idea to get your day off with a good cup of coffee. You can choose your favorite blend – the most important part here is that you enjoy your coffee with no sugar or milk.

After you had your coffee, get your day started. Try to keep yourself active. If you keep busy, you're less likely to think about eating something. You'll keep your mind distracted and yourself on track with your intermittent fasting diet plan. During this time, you should ensure that you drink an adequate amount of water.

As the day goes by, you should try to stay strong. By around 3 pm, if you do feel the hunger coming on, try to drink a sparkling water drink. Aim for one that does not contain any calories. There are various flavored sparkling waters on the market that are available in zero-calorie options. The sparkling water will usually help to make your stomach feel at least a little fuller and can be a great tool for getting yourself through that final push until you can have something to eat.

When the time comes to break your fasting period and start to enjoy food, try to do it slowly. Avoid pushing a 500-gram steak down your throat. Start with something simple, such as a protein bar. There are protein bars that are packed with useful nutrients, along with a high amount of protein, but still low on the calorie part. Consider this a treat – a way to reward yourself for keeping strong and pushing through the entire fasting period.

Wait about an hour and then have a fruit. An apple

is a really great choice in this case. Apples are extremely nutritious, and they taste great – plus they contain a lot of water and apples are low in calories. You can cut the apple into small slices and then enjoy them slice-by-slice. In addition to tasting great, the apple will also give you a burst of energy that should help you get through the period until you are going to have dinner.

If you do feel the need to have another snack before dinner time strikes, try to have some water first. If you feel hungry after the water, then try to aim for a low-calorie snack. Limit yourself to about 100 calories – but only have a snack if it is absolutely necessary. Perhaps have another fruit.

Try to prepare dinner so that you can enjoy it at around 6.30pm to 7.00pm. Dinner can be big, but should still consist of healthy food choices. There is no use in trying to take advantage of the benefits that intermittent fasting has for your well-being when you are just going to smack a McDonald's burger down your throat the moment you get a chance to eat.

Perhaps prepare some brown rice with chicken, or maybe some home-made meatballs with spaghetti. Try to include some vegetables as well. There is no need to limit yourself to just one or two different meals. There are thousands of recipes all over the internet that you can enjoy – just be sure that there are not too many calories in the meal and ensure the ingredients are good for you.

Before you go to bed, aim to get a few more calories into your body. At around 10 pm, you can treat yourself with a little snack. Aim for some-thing that is below around 400 calories to avoid stuffing your body with a lot of calories just before you go to sleep. A good idea at this time would be a bar or a cookie, or anything else that contains a high amount of protein.

Example #2

Let's take a look at another example of how you can use the intermittent fasting program to help you reach your specific goals. In this example, we are going to consider those who are only starting out with intermittent fasting and still find that it is incredibly difficult to make the adjustment that is needed. Thus, the fasting window will only last for 14 hours per day, instead of 16, and the eating window is extended to 10 hours, instead of only eight hours.

Planning Your Meals for Specific Goals

The example meal plan discussed above is a good option if you are trying to lose weight, but not all people who are opting for an intermittent fasting diet will want to lose weight. At the beginning of this book, we dis-cussed the various benefits that this type of eating plan could have – so there are other reasons why people are choosing to follow an intermit-tent fasting diet as well.

You will need to take such factors into account.

For example, let's say you want to bulk up and gain some lean muscle mass while you are following a diet that takes advantage of intermittent fasting – you will need to aim at increasing your intake of calories through the periods in which you are allowed to eat. This can be quite difficult since the window can be somewhat small.

If you go about this all in a smart way, then you will be able to achieve an ideal number of calories during the day, and you will gain enough protein and other nutrients to support your body, as well as reach your goal of bulking up.

There are many high-protein foods that you can include in your diet and consume them throughout your eating window. Try out some Greek yogurt, or perhaps cook up some cheese quesadilla. A single serving of cheese quesadilla contains around 10 grams worth of protein. A serving of Greek yogurt can offer you about 13 grams of protein. There are many different options – try to be creative and find ways to integrate these protein-rich foods into your meal plan.

Calculating Your Daily Macro Requirements

When it comes to following a diet, it is always useful to calculate your specific daily macro requirements in order to know how much food you should consume, and the specific types of food you should ideally consume. There are three macros that you will need to focus on – this includes proteins, fats, and, of course, carbohydrates.

In most cases, whether you are trying to recompose your body, lose weight, or gain muscle mass, you will focus on achieving a relatively high protein intake. On some days, your fat intake will be lower than others. Carbohydrate intake should always make up for the remaining calories that are left after you have determined the amount of protein and fat to consume in your daily diet.

You will generally also have different macro requirements for days when you will be training, compared to those days where you will not be training and will rather take a resting day instead.

Determine Your Daily Caloric Intake Requirement.

Before we can discuss how your daily macro requirements can be calculated, we first need to look at how you can determine the most ideal number of calories that you should consume each day.

There are different strategies that can be used to help you determine your ideal daily caloric requirements. Below, we will use a basic system known as the "Harris-Benedict formula" to help you determine the best number of calories that you should consume. I will lay this out in a step-by-step manner to make things easier for you:

1.   The first step is to calculate your BMR. This is a figure that is generally considered the number of calories that your body will re-quire to survive if you are physically inactive – particularly when you might be in a coma. This really is a two step process, so follow both of the steps I outline below:

a. Calculate your Lean Body Mass with the following formula -> LBM = weight – (weight * (body fat percentage / 100)).

b. Calculate your BMR with the following formula -> BMR = 370 + 21.6 * LBM (Note: LBM / Lean Body Mass should be in kilograms)

2. Next, you will need to make a couple of adjustments to your BMR. Start by considering your physical activity level. The more physically active you are, the more you will need to eat on a day-to-day basis. Follow the following formulas to calculate your TDEE.

a. If you do not exercise much and live a sedentary lifestyle, then the formula is 1.2 x BMR

b. If you participate in light activities up to three times per week, then the formula is 1.375 x BMR

c. If you are moderately active and participate in physical activity up to five days per week, then the formula is 1.55 x BMR

d. If you are very active and take part in training programs or sports for seven days per week, then the formula is 1.725 x BMR

e. If you are extremely active and participate in heavy workouts multiple times each day, then the formula is 1.9 x BMR

3. Once you have calculated your TDEE, the next part of the process is to consider your specific goals. There are three particularly popular

goals that people often strive toward when they consider implementing intermittent fasting. This includes fat loss, muscle gain, and body recomposition. The specific goal that you are striving to will have an impact on how you should adjust your daily caloric consumption as follow:

a.   If you want to gain muscle mass, then add 20% to the TDEE you calculated previously.

b.   If you want to lose weight, then you need to consider your current body fat percentage. Follow this guide to understand how much you should reduce your caloric intake in order to achieve your goal:

   i.   Body fat percentage of 30% or higher -> reduce daily calorie intake by 30%

   ii.   Body fat percentage between 20% and 30% -> reduce daily calorie intake by 25%

   iii.   Body fat percentage between 10% and 20% -> re-duce daily calorie intake by 20%

   iv.   Body fat percentage under 10% -> reduce daily calorie intake by 15%

c.   If you want to recomposition your body, then do not make any adjustments to your daily caloric intake.

Now that you have an idea of the average daily caloric intake you should achieve to reach your goals through intermittent fasting, there is an important step left – caloric intake should defer on training days and resting days.

It is generally recommended to have a 40%

different between these days.

• On your resting days, you should follow this formula to determine how many calories you should consume: calculated daily calorie in-take x 0.8

• On training days where you will participate in physical activities, follow this formula: calculated daily calorie intake x 1.2

Calculating Your Ideal Macros

Now that you know how many calories you need to consume on specific days of the week, the next step would be to calculate the ideal amount of each macro that should make up your diet.

I usually start by setting my own protein intake level – protein should be kept high as it is the building block for your muscles. In addition to protein's effect on muscles, this is also a satiating macro, which means you'll feel fuller when the majority of your meal consists of protein.

It is generally recommended to calculate your protein intake based on your lean body mass, with a recommendation between 2.3 and 3.1 grams of protein per one kilogram of body weight. For me, the ideal amount is 2.5 grams of protein per kilogram body weight, but each person is different. If this amount does not work for you, then adjust your protein intake accordingly.

Fat intake is usually also calculated based on your lean body mass. The recommended range is between 0.9 and 1.3 grams of fat per one kilogram of body weight. Make sure that you gain fat from healthy sources and not from takeaway French fries!

When you deduct the number of calories in the fat and protein sources that you will be consuming, the remainder should be filled with carbohydrates. Each one gram of carbohydrates will give you a total of four calories.

CHAPTER 7

TIPS FOR GETTING STARTED WITH INTERMITTENT FASTING

Most people who are used to their daily routine of having three meals and never skipping out will find it intimidating to get started with implementing intermittent fasting into their lives. This especially goes for those individuals who eat multiple times a day and who have a particularly hard time controlling their cravings. With intermittent fasting, it is vital that you stick to your schedule for maximum benefits. That said, there is no need to act like you are in a military camp.

With some simple steps, you can make the entire process of adopting intermittent fasting a fun journey for yourself – an experimental procedure that will take some time to perfect, but once you get there, you will be able to master this technique and gain many health benefits. Keep this in mind when you feel like quitting – you will only be able to reach that goal if you keep yourself motivated at all times.

Before you jump into intermittent fasting, you might want to take some things into consideration first. In particular, if you have been diagnosed with any type of chronic disease and if you are taking medications, then you should first talk with your physician to determine if this is a safe option for you.

Furthermore, don't overcomplicate things. Start small. Break the process up into small steps. Reach for smaller goals and ultimately aim for that big goal of fully implementing fasting techniques into your life. If you cave or something goes wrong, do not let it get you down. Instead, just keep on going.

Here Is a Step-By-Step Guide to Help You Out.

The first step is to determine what type of technique you want to adopt. The 16/8 is highly recommended for beginners. What you may not know is that you are already halfway there. You are fasting while you are sleeping – we bet you haven't thought of this before… Now, to get to the 16/8, you will simply have to start skipping breakfast, for example.

Decide on the time slots – dedicate eating windows and fasting windows. If you follow the 16/8 plan, for example, you can decide to have your first meal of the day at lunchtime, instead of early in the morning, and finish off at 8 PM, for example. Give yourself a good 16 hours without food – this would include your seven to nine hours of sleep, which you should be getting to keep your body healthy.

Start small and simple – try this for one day and see if you can make it. If you feel like you run out of energy too quickly, then stretch your eating window a little and make your fasting window narrower. As the days go by, start to shorten your eating window and make your fasting window longer – that is until you can go without food for 16 hours at a time. If you make a mistake by giving in to the temptation of having a snack when the hunger becomes extreme, don't beat yourself up over it. Simply start over.

In addition to deciding on the perfect option for you, it is also a good idea to consider why you want to include intermittent fasting in your life. When you are doing this for a specific purpose, then you will have some-thing to keep you motivated. Perhaps you want to lose weight. This is a great reason to fast – remember we looked at scientific evidence before that supported the weight loss advantages of intermittent fasting...

If you want simply want to help prolong your lifespan and reduce your risk of certain diseases, then these are also important reasons. Write them down if you have to – on your schedule. This will keep you motivated to ensure you can reach your goal.

Apps and Tools That Will Make Your Journey Easier

Things can become confusing, especially at first, when you start with intermittent fasting. This is why using some essential tools to help you keep track of everything would be a good idea. You can always go old school and decide to plot down your schedule on a piece of paper. Perhaps buy a new notebook that is dedicated to this journey you are about to go on. Write down your schedule and mark down your progress. This will also help you go back and track your performance, as well as see where you have slipped up – giving you the ability to identify opportunities for improvement in the future.

If you rather prefer to keep things digital, then try out a couple of intermittent fasting apps. You would be surprised at how many there are. Take a look at some – they are available on both Google Play Store and Apple Store. Consider the user reviews. Then decide on an app that you like – and try to use it every day to help you keep track of your journey.

LIFE is currently one of the top-rated apps used for this purpose. It gives you the ability to record data for any type of intermittent fasting method that you would like to follow. You can easily adjust your schedule, and the app will even tell you when your body is expected to be in the ketosis phase. To keep you inspired and motivated, the app also allows you to join groups of other people who are on the same journey as you are.

CHAPTER 8

WHO SHOULD AVOID INTERMITTENT FASTING?

While intermittent fasting is generally considered a safe and effective lifestyle decision and a way of eating, there are some cases where this particular diet may not be the most appropriate option for a person. It is important that individuals who are interested in adopting an intermittent fasting diet first consider the pros and cons of this diet, and take a look at the specific risks that have been associated with this way of eating. If the individual finds that they might fall within the risky side of things, then intermittent fasting may not be an ideal option for them. In such cases, the person may be better off opting for an alternative diet that can help them achieve their specific goals.

As with any type of meal plan and adjustment to

how you are eating, it can be beneficial to first consult with a physician on intermittent fasting before you start to implement such a plan into your own life. It is best to choose a physician that already knows you and your medical history – this way, and the physician will be able to determine if you would be a good candidate for intermittent fasting and if a different type of diet might be more appropriate for you.

Women should especially ensure they consult with their physician before they decide to start following an intermittent fasting diet. The reason for this is because intermittent fasting has been found to have an adverse impact on the hormonal balance within a woman's body in some cases. When a woman's hormones are not in balance, then she may experience a number of potential adverse effects.

Some potential adverse events that a woman may experience when her hormones are out of balance may include:

• Developing skin-related problems. Dry skin is quite common amongst women who have an imbalance in hormones within their body. Another very common issue that this particular problem may cause is the development of pimples. Skin discolorations may also occur in some cases. These can all cause a woman to experience problems in terms of their mental health – they may start to feel self-conscious about their appearance.

• Brain fog may also develop when a woman's hormones are out of balance. This can be an extremely dreadful issue, as the woman may find that they are unable to focus and concentrate, and their memory may also be adversely affected. In turn, the woman will experience a significant decline in their productivity. With this in mind, their time at work will be less effective.

• In addition to brain fog, many women find that they develop fatigue – often quite frequently – with an imbalance in their hormone levels. Fatigue can be just as dreadful. The woman may find that she feels tired all the time and wants to sleep a lot.

• Mood swings are also relatively common among women with issues in terms of their hormonal balance. Along with the mood swings may come sessions of anxiety and stress, as well as depression.

• In some cases, a woman may also find that their libido becomes low with inadequate regulation of their hormones. With a low libido, the woman will not be interested in participating in sexual inter-course with their partner.

People who are suffering from certain conditions will also need to be careful when it comes to implementing an intermittent fasting plan into their life. Some of the conditions that are considered risk factors for experiencing adverse effects when it comes to intermittent fasting include adrenal fatigue, existing hormonal issues, and gastrointestinal problems. Furthermore, people who have a history of eating disorders are also ad-vised to avoid intermittent fasting as this may yield unpleasant results potentially.

CHAPTER 9

THE SCIENTIFIC EVIDENCE BEHIND INTERMITTENT FASTING

When it comes to learning more about specific types of diet plans and lifestyle habits, it is always important to take a look at the scientific re-search behind such programs. With this in mind, the same applies to those who are interested in taking on an intermittent fasting plan – whether it is to lose weight or to build muscle mass or to enjoy a healthy way of living simply and to experience the benefits. If you are interested in intermittent fasting, be sure to first take a good look at the scientific evidence behind this eating plan. Do not only consider the potential benefits that intermittent fasting might have for you, but also consider the possible side-effects and downsides that may apply to those who are following a diet that is based on intermittent fasting.

Many scientific studies have been done on intermittent fasting, which can help you determine the efficiency and safety of this particular diet pro-gram. In this chapter, I would like to go over a few of the previous studies that have been conducted.

"Daily fasting works for weight loss, finds the report on 16:8 diet." *https://www.sciencedaily.com/releases/2018/0 6/180618113038.htm*

The University of Illinois at Chicago published the results of a recent study they conduct, titled Daily fasting works for weight loss, finds the report on 16:8 diet. The study was officially published on ScienceDaily on the 18th of June, 2018.

The study focused on obtaining data relevant to the effects of intermit-tent fasting on the body weight of individuals who are obese. There was a total of 23 volunteers who participated in the study. All of the volunteers were obese, with a BMI that measured 35 or higher. The average age of the participants was about 45.

During the study, the participants were asked to consume their meals be-tween 10 am in the morning and 6 pm at night During the rest of the day, the participant was asked to undergo a fast – where they were not al-lowed to consume any type of food or beverages, except for water and selected beverages that do not contain calories. This particular study lasted for a total of 12 weeks.

Several benefits were noted by the scientists who

were involved in the study. The results that were obtained in this study were compared to results from a previous study that also focused on the effects of fasting on obesity and body weight, but that previous study did not implement time-restricted fasting protocols.

In particular, this study found that weight loss was much more significant among those individuals who followed an intermittent fasting diet plan. Calorie consumption was also reduced by a statistically significant level. In addition to the weight-related benefits, it was also found that the study participants experienced an improvement in their blood pressure levels. With obesity being linked to high blood pressure – and this condition, in turn, associated with a range of adverse effects in the body, including blood vessel damage, this is certainly a benefit that needs to be noted.

The average participant in this particular study was found to consume 350 calories less than they did before they started to follow the intermit-tent fasting diet that was presented to them by the researchers involved in the study. Additionally, the individuals involved in the study were also found to lose an average of 3% of their total body weight. Additionally, systolic blood pressure levels were decreased by an average of seven millimeters per mercury, or mm Hg.

Scientists involved in the study concluded by saying that the obese population should know that there are ways that they can lose weight effectively without the need for excessively starving themselves, without having to count calories to the last digit, and without the need to eliminate all of the most tasteful foods that they are used to consuming.

It should be noted that results in this particular study on intermittent fasting and the diet's effect on weight loss had similar results compared to the previous studies that focused on fasting in general in terms of insulin resistance, cholesterol regulation, and fat mass. Still, this holds important evidence that intermittent fasting can be a good tool in a person's weight loss strategy.

"Intermittent fasting interventions for the treatment of overweight and obesity in adults."

A study conducted scientists at the University of Glasgow in the United Kingdom, published on the 1st of February 2018, looked at how intermit-tent fasting could be utilized as an intervention in the treatment of excessive weight among adults in the local region. The study was conducted in such a way to compare the results obtained with intermittent fasting to the results that can be achieved through no treatment, as well as through more traditional means of treating obesity in adult patients.

All of the patients who were part of the study had a BMI that was more than 25, which classifies them as being overweight. A large number of the study participants were obese as well, which means their BMI was higher than 30. All of the participants were over the age of 18 at the time of the study.

Each patient who participated in the study were provided with a diet plan that they had to follow. On intermittent fasting days, the patient was ad-vised to consume a diet that resulted in less than 800 kcal in total consumption per day. The study lasted for 12 weeks in total to ensure adequate time for results to be achieved, as it is known that appropriate weight loss results with any changes in diet can take a while.

The most significant results noted by this study were the reduction in the body weight of the participants who were involved in the intermittent fasting diet. In addition to these primary outcomes of the study, there were several secondary outcomes that the scientists who were involved in the study noted as well.

The secondary outcomes presented by the study was divided into multiple groups, and consists of:

- Anthropometric outcomes: Participants had a lower BMI at the end of the study and smaller waist circumference. Fat mass and fat-free mass were also reduced significantly, compared to the other studies that were compared to the results obtained from the intermittent fasting programs.

- Cardio-metabolic outcomes: Blood glucose levels were improved, along with insulin levels. The study also noted statistically significant improvements in the blood pressure levels of patients who participated in the intermittent fasting program. Lipoprotein pro-files had also improved.

It should be noted that some results obtained in the intermittent fasting study were very similar to the results that were obtained in the other studies that these results were compared to.

In the end, this is yet another study that provides evidence of the effective results that intermittent fasting can provide a person with if they follow through on the particular plan that has been developed for them. Dedication and patience are two key factors to ensure the individual following this type of diet is able to achieve success and reach the goals they have set out for themselves.

"Intermittent Fasting with or without Exercise Prevents Weight Gain and Improves Lipids in Diet-Induced Obese Mice"
https://www.ncbi.nlm.nih.gov/pmc/articles/PMC5872764/

While many people tend to exclude animal-based studies when they are looking for evidence on a specific topic, it is important to consider the fact that these animal-studies pave an important way for future human studies to be implemented. Thus, I would like us to take a look at one particular study in the MDPI Nutrients Journal, published on the 12th of March 2018. The study looked at how intermittent fasting would affect the potential of gaining weight, as well as the lipid profiles, in mice that were purposely made obese through a specific diet that they were fed.

In this study, laboratory rats were fed a diet that was high in sugar and fat for 24 weeks in total. The diet was induced upon them at the age of eight weeks. After the 24-week period had concluded, the mice were divided into five appropriate groups in order to gain a more accurate insight into how beneficial intermittent fasting would be for weight loss, the prevention of weight gain, and more.

These five groups consisted of the following:
- Baseline control
- No intervention
- Intermittent Fasting
- High-intensity interval training, or HIIT
- Combination group, which included both high-intensity interval training and intermittent fasting protocols.

Several factors were taken into account during this study. The body com-position and general strength of each mouse were analyzed, along with a number of blood variables. Measurements were taken before the study was officially started, as well as at week 10 and at week 12.

The groups that had intermittent fasting included in their program all experienced a significant reduction in weight gain, even when fed a diet that induced obesity. Fat accumulation in these groups was also much lower than in the groups that did not include intermittent fasting. In addition to these benefits, the scientists that were in charge of the study al-so noted that the lipoprotein levels in the laboratory rats (in particular, their LDL cholesterol) were reduced significantly as well.

These results were observed in the group of mice that were simply placed on an intermittent fasting program, as well as those who had an intermit-tent fasting program along with high-intensity interval training.

The conclusion of the study was that intermittent fasting could result in assistance to reduce the risk of excess weight gain. The diet can also be useful for reducing fat accumulation in the body and may also be useful for improving cholesterol balance. These results can be achieved even when intermittent fasting is implemented without an active exercise plan, according to the evidence presented by this study.

Further research is still needed among human subjects to determine if similar effects can be achieved since laboratory rats were utilized in this particular study.

"Intermittent Fasting And Human Metabolic Health"
https://www.ncbi.nlm.nih.gov/pmc/articles/PMC4516560/

Instead of focusing solely on the weight loss benefits that intermittent fasting has to offer, one study, led by the University of California, rather decided to focus on how intermittent fasting would benefit the entire metabolic system of the human body. Instead of doing a separate study, however, the group of researchers who compiled this publication decided to take a look at various existing studies in order to gain an overview of how this diet has affected participants of various studies in the past – and to then make a conclusion as to what health benefits should really be associated with intermittent fasting.

A variety of studies were included in this research project, and their data have been individually reported in the published paper. Below is a quick overview of the data that has been presented here:

- Halberg 2005 study: Eight male patients participated, all of whom were healthy, and none of them were obese. Alternate day fasting techniques were used, with 20-hour fasting windows. The study was conducted over a period of 15 days. Blood glucose levels were significantly reduced by the end of the study. Adiponectin levels rose, and leptin levels were also observed to be much lower than at the start of the study.

- Heilbronn 2005 study: A total of 16 patients participated, half male and half female. All patients were at a healthy weight. The study was conducted over a period of 22 days. There were 36-hour fasting intervals introduced to participants of the study. Insulin levels were significantly reduced at the end of the study.

- Horne 2012 study: There were 30 participants in the study. Twenty of the participants were female, and the rest were male. All participants were over the age of 18 and healthy. The study was only con-ducted over a period of one single day. Participants were asked to fast for a period of 28 hours, in which they were only advised to consume water. Levels of both LDL cholesterol and HDL cholesterol were increased, while triglyceride levels were observed to be lower by the end of the fasting period. Glucose and insulin levels were also significantly reduced, which provided beneficial effects for individuals with diabetes. There was also a slight decrease in the weight of the individuals who participated in the study.

- Johnson 2007 study: Only 10 participants were included in the study. A total of eight were female, and two were male. All of the patients had asthma and were considered overweight, but not obese. The study was conducted over a period of eight weeks. At the end of the study, body weight was reduced among the participants. There was an increase in HDL cholesterol and a reduction in triglycerides. Two inflammatory markers were also reduced, including BDNF and TNF-a.

- Varady 2009 study: A total of 20 participants were involved in this particular study, with 12 being female and the rest male. The study was conducted over eight weeks, and only obese individuals were involved in the study. Participants experienced a reduction in their body weight, as well as lower triglyceride levels and LDL cholesterol levels.

CHAPTER 10

FREQUENTLY ASKED QUESTIONS ABOUT INTERMITTENT FASTING

Can I drink coffee while I am fasting?

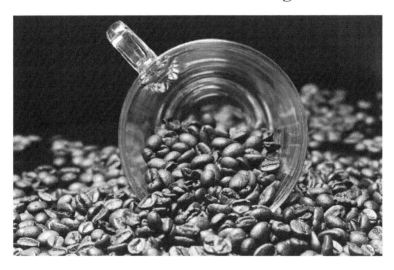

Coffee is a beverage that millions of people enjoy each and every day. This is why many people are concerned that they might have to give up their cup of coffee that they enjoy so much each morning if they are going to start following an intermittent fasting plan – the majority of these plans will tell you to sustain from eating until later in the afternoon and to skip on breakfast for a boost in benefits.

Fortunately, there is no need to worry if you are planning to implement intermittent fasting into your diet – and would still like to have a cup or two of coffee in the morning. There is, however, one particular factor that you do need to note here. If you want to have a cup of coffee after waking up and your intermittent fasting plan demands that you continue with your fasting window in the morning, then it means no sugar and no milk for you. While some people have noted that it is okay to add one splash of milk to your coffee while fasting, this is usually not recommended if you are serious about losing weight while you are following an intermittent fasting plan.

Coffee can actually be a great addition to your diet plan and be a good boost for getting through that last period of fasting. When you opt for a cup of coffee in the morning, you will get an energy boost – and since the caffeine in coffee may provide you with benefits for as long as six hours, you can easily glide on these effects until the time comes to break your fasting period.

Coffee has also been shown to speed up metabolism, which is great for anyone looking to lose weight. You'll end up burning even more fat.

Additionally, coffee will help to keep your mind

sharp during the morning and avoid those dreadful times when brain fog hits you because you are running on empty.

There is another benefit that should be noted in terms of having a cup of coffee for breakfast, instead of indulging in a big breakfast. This particular benefit comes in handy for those who are looking to work out while they are still fasting – many people prefer a morning workout, after all. There are some people who follow an intermittent fasting plan that finds they do not have the same level of energy while working out compared to eating a good breakfast before they go out and hit the gym. When you drink some coffee, you'll get a boost in both physical performances, and cognitive function – both of these are crucial for a good workout in the gym.

Should I break my fast with a big or small meal?

Another popular question that people tend to ask when it comes to intermittent fasting is how exactly they should break their fast. The opinions in regards to breaking a fasting window while following an intermit-tent fasting program is mixed. Some suggest that you break the fast with a big meal that is packed with calories to load your body with protein and other essential nutrients, while others suggest that you start out simple and small, and then gradually work up to that big meal.

There really isn't a single perfect answer to this question, but it should be taken into account that when breaking a fast, the body is still in a fat burning mode. When you hit your body with too many calories at once, you can switch off this mode and experience less of the benefits that you are expecting from your intermittent fasting plan.

Thus, it is generally not considered a good idea to break your fast with a meal that is considered loaded in calories. I personally find that it is much more convenient to start things out slowly. Perhaps break that fasting period with a green salad, or perhaps some Greek yogurt. There are many options that can help to satisfy the hunger you have built up during the fast, offer you a series of healthy and essential nutrients, but without causing your metabolism to shut down.

After the fast has been broken and you have had your first meal, plan for a second and a third meal as well. Be sure that these meals will also be nutritious and healthy. I enjoy a big meal that makes up most of the calories I should consume daily by the end of the day. Some might prefer this "big meal" to happen in between their first and third meal – this way, they can start their eating cycle and end the cycle with something small. This would also help to reduce the number of calories you should consume just before you go to bed.

If you are not sure which one you prefer, be sure to consider the various meal plan examples that I have shared with you in this book. You'll find a couple of different meal plans spread out throughout this book – they are all great for those who are starting out without knowing which type of meal plan they would like to implement with their intermittent fasting program.

A good idea would also be to experiment with different options. Try to make the second meal of the eating period your big meal of the day. See how your body reacts. You might also try the first and the final meal of the day – make these your big meals. Really observe how you feel with each of these options. You'll eventually start to notice that your body re-acts better to one of these particular options – or perhaps spreading out your calories equally. When you find the right option, continue with it.

How do I cope with my hunger during the fasting window?

When you are starting out with intermittent fasting for the first time and you are used to eating three or more meals a day, along with some snacking in-between, then there really is no doubt that for the initial period of intermittent fasting, you will experience hunger and some cravings. This is something that most people struggle with – and it is an issue that often causes people to give up on intermittent fasting and either return to their usual way of eating or turn to another type of diet to help them possibly lose the excess weight that is causing them concern.

The key to success in terms of coping with hunger when starting with an intermittent fasting program really is patience. You will need to have patience when it comes to feeling the effects of this diet come into play. It will take some time, but when you push through these hunger strikes, then you will start to notice the cravings become fewer and fewer as the days go by. Instead of experiencing cravings for candy and other un-healthy foods, you will start to experience hunger – this is a good thing, so do not think of the hunger as a bad thing that is striking you at the most unpleasant times.

Since you are not craving unhealthy foods, you will be less likely to start searching for donuts and candy bars to snack on. You'll also find that it is easier to push through until you reach the time where you can have your first meal.

If you do feel that you are unable to cope anymore and those last few hours simply seem too far away, then have sparkling water. This will help to make your stomach feel full for a little while – in turn, and you will find that it becomes much easier to last for an hour or two more in order to reach the time when you can finally break your fast.

How will I train if I am running empty on food?

While coping with hunger is one thing that people struggle with when they are following an intermittent fasting plan, another issue that some also find is that they are not sure how they will continue with their training regimen once they start to follow this type of program. The obvious idea behind intermittent fasting is that you would find yourself running low on food just in the nick of time when you decide to hit the gym – this means you do not have an adequate source of fuel to give you that energy you need to push through the entire session.

In reality, some people actually find that they are able to train more efficiently when their stomach is not full. There are also many who have claimed training during a fasting period is more beneficial – and that it is sometimes even easier.

If you do feel that you are unable to get through that upcoming training session because you feel "empty" and out of energy, then perhaps con-sider opting for a cup of coffee – no milk or sugar, however. The coffee will give you the boost you need to get through the entire session and may even give you some energy afterward to last until the time at which you can break the fast.

Keep in mind that when training on an empty stomach, your body will not have food to turn to in order to generate energy. In turn, this also means that your body will start to turn to the fat storages within your body in order to generate the energy that you need to continue running on that treadmill or to continue pushing those weights. This, in turn, also means fat is burnt faster and much more effectively.

Is it okay to cheat now-and-then?

When it comes to intermittent fasting for weight loss, people are usually inclined to follow a specific meal plan and diet that will give them guidance on what they can eat during the periods that they are allowed to consume calories. In the majority of cases, diets will be somewhat restricted – they will usually include healthy foods that are relatively low in carbohydrates while being high in protein and other essential nutrients.

The healthy meals will surely make you feel great, but there is no shame in wanting to have a "cheat" snack or even a cheat meal now-and-then. The big question now is whether or not it is okay for you to have a cheat day, or even just a cheat snack or treat.

In reality, having a "cheat" day will not do you a lot of harm in terms of your weight loss results – the important part here is to ensure that this does not happen every day. Try to limit yourself to a cheat once a week at most. Perhaps grab a bar of chocolate from your local supermarket or, if you really want to go bigger, get your family to agree to dinner at a local restaurant.

When you do have a cheat day or meal, it is important that you take the calories consumed while 'cheating' into account. This number of calories you will have to make up for the next day – this way, you'll continue to experience the benefits of the diet.

Consider the number of calories you went over your daily limit today – perhaps that bar of chocolate added another 150 calories to your day.

The next day, be sure to reduce your calorie consumption to make up for the excess in calories that you decided to have the previous day.

https://www.ncbi.nlm.nih.gov/pmc/articles/PMC4516560/

CHAPTER 11

CONCLUSION

I hope this book helped you understand the basics of occasional fasting and the benefits that this diet will bring into your life. By practicing occasionally fasting while you are fit, without having to adhere to strict diets that can be harmful to your health, you will succeed in reducing weight and be in the best form of your life.

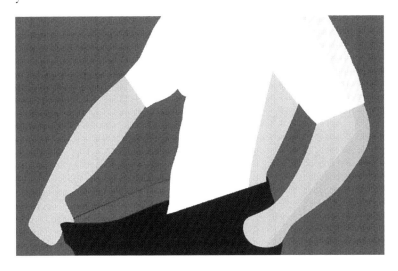

Understanding the principles of occasional fasting, will not only help to reduce your weight, but it will also contribute to the strengthening of your mental health by training your brain to be durable and to resist food in moments that are meant for fasting. This way you will become a stronger person. But the psyche is not the only thing that will be strengthened. Who does not want strong and well-shaped muscles? Well, occasional fasting will help in creating this. You must be wondering how can something that deprives you of food, helps you build muscle when you know that building muscle requires more calorie intake. Well, this is not the case. Basically, intermittent fasting will teach you to appreciate food and to refer to a healthy diet that will become part of your everyday life. With the right combination of fat, carbohydrates, protein, fresh fruits and vegetables, you will able to create meals that the body needs on the days of not fasting.

The next step is to list all the various methods of intermittent fasting once more, to help you choose the one that will best suit your lifestyle and daily responsibilities, and gradually start to change your life and take care of your health forever. Of course, do not be alarmed if you are suddenly unable to endure the whole fasting period. Allow your body some time to get used to this way of eating, and over time you will be able to lengthen the time for fasting. Combine some simple exercises to increase the burning of fat from your body, or prepare your own exercise plan that will fit your fitness level. But, try not to forget the recommendations given in the book of the combination of the intensity of exercise on the days when you are fasting and the days when you are not fasting.

It is important to plan exercise days well. If you practice high-intensity workouts on the fasting day, you will feel exhausted, and your muscles will be under a lot of stress, which is not good when you are trying to shape and enhance. Also, to get those well established and toned muscles, drink plenty of water (at least eight glasses, but really this is the mini-mum amount we need) and remember to combine protein, carbohydrates, and fat before and after training to help your muscles grow. Take the recommendations for gradual entry into the process of fasting and become one step closer to changing your whole life and becoming happier and satisfied with your visual appearance and health.

References

https://www.webmd.com/diet/obesity/obesity-health-risks#1

https://www.healthline.com/nutrition/warrior-diet-guide

https://www.medicalnewstoday.com/articles/321486.php

https://www.sciencedaily.com/releases/2018/06/180618113038.htm

https://insights.ovid.com/crossref?an=01938924-201802000-00016

https://www.ncbi.nlm.nih.gov/pmc/articles/PMC5872764/

https://www.ncbi.nlm.nih.gov/pmc/articles/PMC4516560/

http://siimland.com/what-can-you-drink-while-fasting/

https://www.bodyandsoul.com.au/nutrition/nutrition-tips/is-coffee-okay-to-drink-while-fasting/news-story/6c3b48475e5150e74558bfef02ee01ef

Made in the USA
Columbia, SC
24 April 2019